CHIDI ANSLEM ADIM

A – Z OF DIVINE HEALTH

26 Keys To Living In Divine Health From A to Z

TABLE OF CONTENTS

DEDICATION

To the Almighty God, the great Healer, for my unfailing health, and for giving me the potential and the grace to put together this book.

To the love of my life, my darling wife, Loveleen, who is my personal source of encouragement and inspiration, for giving me the 'push' I needed to start and finish this work.

To millions of people trapped in sickness by Satan's lies about divine healing.

To millions of people, around the world, lying critically sick, robbed of the health and vitality to maximize and fulfill their God given potentials.

To everyone that will go beyond healing to living in divine health through the teachings of this book.

INTRODUCTION

The need for this book especially at this time that nations of the world are plagued with different sicknesses and diseases cannot be overemphasized.

God created a perfect world and then created man in His image and likeness to share in His divine nature. God put His perfect creature, man in a spectacular beautiful Garden, Eden, to care for it. God gave man authority and dominion over the earth and everything in it.

The instructions of God was simple, dress and keep the Garden, eat freely from every tree of the garden, but stay away from the tree of the knowledge of good and evil. The day you eat it, you will surely die.

Before God ever created man and put him in the garden, there was Lucifer who became the devil when he rebelled against God. The devil wanted the authority and dominion God had given to man and was determined to ruin God's creation.

Man committed high treason against God when instead of obeying God; they (Adam and Eve) chose to believe the devil. Satan became man's boss legally, took authority and dominion God gave man, because of the spiritual law that say "you become slave of whatever you chose to obey" (Romans 6:16).

The fall of man and the dominion of Satan ushered in different evil and curses including death, sin, sickness and disease upon all mankind. But God in His infinite love and mercy sent Jesus (the second Adam) to redeem us from the dominion of Satan. By accepting the redemptive provision of God made available in Jesus Christ, we are translated into the kingdom of light, where we can live in total dominion over Satan and every evil he brought including sin, sickness and disease. It is therefore now ignorance that keep people trapped in sickness.

The Bible said in Hosea 4:6 (KJV) that, "My people are destroyed for lack of knowledge." It didn't say, "My people are destroyed because of the devil." The greatest enemy of our well-being and longevity is ignorance of the right keys to living in divine health.

It doesn't matter if you have been diagnosed with a life-threatening illness. Maybe you have been told that you have a terminal disease. Or perhaps you or someone you love is desperately in need of healing. What you need is "A – Z of Divine Health: 26 Keys to living in divine health from A to Z."

This book is a life changer. It reveals powerful keys and truths that if for any reason they enter your heart, they will make you victorious over any sickness or disease. You cannot operate these keys and still be tossed about with one illness or the other. And that is why the enemy will do anything to keep you from standing on such revelation.

Healing is good but divine health is far better. God's will for you is that you live in total and perfect health (3 John 1:2). My life was forever changed the moment I discovered the truth about God's will for healing and the keys to living in divine health in September, 2006. Since then, I have walked day-to-day in divine health, living a sickness free life. You too can walk in divine health.

A - Z of Divine Health is complete, whether it is A for "Accept Jesus and Be Saved", B for "Building Your Faith for Divine Healing", H for "Healing Power of the Holy Spirit", or Z for "Zion, A Place of Absolute Health". The entire alphabets cover how to receive healing, how to keep the healing and how to live day-to-day in health.

In this brief but thorough Bible-based study, I will be exploring it all, showing you 26 keys to living in divine health from A to Z

KEY #1: A – ACCEPT JESUS AND BE SAVED

God is a Spirit, and He created man in His image and likeness, to share in His divine nature, so it was impossible for the God-like man to get sick. However, there was a disruption and man fell from grace. Jesus came to restore man to his lost position. Will you accept Jesus and be saved?

<u>Everything Was Very Good At The Beginning</u>

"And God saw every thing that he had made, and, behold, it was very good..." (Genesis 1:31).

The world we live in today is not the perfect world that God created. Sickness, which obviously does not fall under the description of "very good" was not created. Sin, sickness, disease and everything evil came as a result of the fall of man in the Garden of Eden.

The disobedience of our first parents, Adam and Eve brought several significant changes that affect all of God's creation. The fall of man brought the earth under sin's curse and led to the degeneration of nature whose original condition was perfect. Thorns and thistles, which symbolize evil including death, sickness and suffering, took over.

So many things went wrong with the fall of man. Bacteria, fungi and other microbes originally designed by God to only benefit man, animals and plants underwent mutation and other degenerative processes.

The deterioration of the human body, the decay of the original good condition of nature, the degeneration of microbes, mistakes and poor decisions of (once perfect) man and constant attack from the devil account for the different sickness and diseases which soon became part of human life.

Though not all illnesses result from affliction of the devil, some illnesses are result of living in a fallen world, others are man-made, but because the devil is behind the fall of man, he is the author of all sickness and disease. When you read Deuteronomy 28:61, you will see that God referred to every sickness and every plague as curse, and the origin of curse is sin, and Satan is the author of sin.

The Dominion of Darkness

"Don't you realize that you become the slave of whatever you chose to obey? You can be a slave to sin, which leads to death, or you can choose to obey God, which leads to righteous living" (Romans 6:16 NLT).

Have you ever wondered why God didn't just destroy Satan, instead of allowing him to run rampage all over, causing havoc? Well, God respects laws, and Satan is operating on a legal ground. God is a covenant keeper and He deals with every being, whether spirit or human, including Satan legally.

Before God ever created man and placed him in the Garden of Eden, there was Lucifer, who was God's vice regent, but became the devil when he rebelled against God.

"How art thou fallen from heaven, O Lucifer, son of the morning! How art thou cut down to the ground, which didst weaken the nations!" (Isaiah 14:2).

Satan through rebellion lost his position and his anointing became corrupted. He made himself God enemy and looked for every opportunity to sabotage God's creation.

When God created man in His image and likeness and gave man dominion over all His creation including the earth, and placed him in a spectacularly beautiful Garden, Satan became jealous. He quickly hatched a plan to ruin God's creation. Adam chose to obey Satan and committed high treason against God, and as a result, he lost his dominion and authority to Satan.

Satan, legally, became the god of this world, and Adam became subject to him, because of the spiritual law that states, "you become slave of whatever you chose to obey" (Romans 6:16). Adam lost his authority and dominion over the earth and everything in the earth to Satan, thus bringing the whole of mankind under Satan's dominion. That Adamic authority is what Satan still operates with today, legally.

The New Birth: A Must For Every Man
"Marvel not that I said unto thee, Ye must be born again" (John 3:7).

One word that perfectly describes God is 'LOVE'. Man wilfully disobeyed God, fell from glory and legally became Satan's slave (Romans 3:23, Romans 6:16) but out love He sent a second Adam (Jesus Christ) to redeem man and restore him to glory and his original position of dominion and authority (John 3:16).

Man would therefore need a rebirth under the second Adam to be taken out of the dominion of darkness, and from under Satan's authority.

"Who hath delivered us from the power of darkness, and hath translated us into the kingdom of his dear Son" (Colossians 1:13).

The first key to living in divine health is to accept Jesus and be saved. This is because as long as you are under Satan's dominion, he has legal rights to stop you from being healed or walking in divine health. You must be born again to legally be catapulted into the kingdom of God's dear Son, Jesus. Only then can you resist the devil and he will flee from you (James 1:7). If you are ready to make Jesus Christ the Lord of your life, pray the following prayer sincerely from your heart with faith.

Prayer for Salvation

Dear God, I come to You in the Name of Jesus. Your word says, "... whosoever shall call on the Name of the Lord shall be saved" (Acts 2:21). I am calling on You. I admit that I am a sinner. I have broken Your laws and my sins have separated me from You. I am truly sorry, and I repent. I ask that You forgive me.

I pray and ask Jesus to come into my life and be my Lord and Savior according to Romans 10: 9 – 10 "That if thou shalt confess with thy mouth the Lord Jesus, and shalt believe in thine heart that God hath raised him from the dead, thou shalt be saved. For with the heart man believeth unto righteousness; and with the mouth confession is made unto salvation".

I hereby confess that Jesus is Lord, and I believe in my heart that He died on the cross for me and that on the third day, God raised Him from the dead. I am now a Christian – a born again child of the Almighty God. Hallelujah!

Heaven is rejoicing over you

If you prayed the prayer above sincerely from your heart with faith, congratulations! You are now a born again child of God, a bona fide citizen of God's kingdom.

Right now heaven is rejoicing over you.

Healing is the children's bread (Matthew 15:26), and as a child of God, healing and divine health belong to you legally. It is your birth right to live in total and perfect health! It is your covenant right!

KEY #2: B - BUILDING YOUR FAITH FOR DIVINE HEALING

"Now faith is the substance of things hoped for, the evidence of things not seen" (Hebrews 11:1). It takes faith to receive anything and everything from God. To move anything from the unseen realm of the spirit to the natural sensual realm, faith is required. Faith is the confidence that what we hope for is real and that it will actually happen.

Faith is putting God's integrity to test. Faith gives God the opportunity to prove that He is indeed the Almighty God, and that is why faith pleases Him so much. As the Heritage Singers put it, "God said it, I believed it, that settles it." Faith is the substance of things hoped for.

What is the Substance of Faith?

What exactly is the substance of faith? If faith is believing that what we hoped for will happen, then there has to be something to hold unto, an evidence for what we hoped for.

Think of it this way: flour is the substance of cake we hope for, it is the primary ingredient which defines what a cake is made of. We need flour to produce cake in the same way we need faith to produce healing. But what is the substance of faith?

The Bible says in Hebrews 11:3, "Through faith we understand that the worlds were framed by the word of God, so that things which are seen were not made of things which do appear." God created the world through faith, and the substance He used was His word. In the beginning of creation, when God created heaven and earth, there was darkness upon the face of the deep. God needed light and He had faith that the light He hoped for will come to be. Again, He used the substance of faith - His word: "And God said, Let there be light: and there was light" (Genesis 1:3).

The substance of faith, the evidence for what we hoped for, the proof of our healing is based on the word of God on healing. Faith for healing and divine health is trust, assurance and confidence in God and His word on healing and divine health.

<u>Why Should I Trust God to keep His Word</u>

"Trust the LORD with all your heart; do not depend on your own understanding" (Proverbs 3:5 NLT). To trust God means to believe in His word and to obey Him. It means to put all our hope in His promises even when everything around us tells us not to trust Him. Why should I trust God to keep His word? Here are ten reasons to trust God to keep His promises.

1. God's word is true:

"Sanctify them through thy truth: thy word is truth" (John 17:17).

It does not matter what anyone or situation say, God's word is the truth.

2. God does not lie:

"God is not a man, so he does not lie. He is not human, so he does not change his mind. Has he ever spoken and failed to act? Has he ever promised and not carried it through?" (Numbers 23:19 NLT).

God values His word even above all His Names, because He is a God of integrity. He says what He means and means everything He says. He has never lied to anyone and He will never lie.

3. God is Just:

"He is the Rock; his deeds are perfect. Everything he does is just and fair. He is a faithful God who does no wrong; how just and upright he is!" (Deuteronomy 32:4 NLT)

You can rely on God because He is Just and everything He does is fair. He wants the very best for us.

4. God has never failed to fulfill His Word:

"Not a single one of all the good promises the Lord had given to the family of Israel was left unfulfilled; everything he had spoken came true" (Joshua 21:45 NLT).

"So shall my word be that goes out from my mouth; it shall not return to me empty, but it shall accomplish that which I purpose, and shall succeed in the thing for which I sent it" (Isaiah 55:11 ESV).

God promised Abraham and Serah a child even when

they were already old and Serah was barren and past the age of child bearing. He fulfilled His promise to them.

God said He will deliver the children of Israel from the hands of the Egyptians, and He did.

He promised to send Jesus to redeem us, He did. He is the unchangeable and He will fulfill all His promises to you too.

5. God is forever faithful:

Another reason why you should trust God to keep His word is because He is faithful even in our unfaithfulness. His faithfulness does not depend on ours. He is true to His word and promises.

"If we are faithless, He remains faithful, for He cannot deny Himself" (2 Timothy 2:13 NASB).

6. God is able:

"And being fully persuaded that, what he had promised, he was able also to perform" (Romans 4:21).

If I make you a promise today, you can be sure I will fulfill it, if I had in the past fulfilled my promises to you. Another thing you will likely consider is whether I have the capacity to fulfill the new promise.

If a man who cannot afford a bicycle Tyre promise you a brand new car, you will not take his word serious, not because he lacks integrity but because he lacks the capacity to fulfill the promise.

If a man makes you a promise, you cannot be certain he will fulfill it because of unforeseen circumstances beyond his control that that may arise.

If God however makes you a promise, be rest assured that He will fulfill it because He is able and there is no impossibility with Him. He is the Almighty and the All-sufficient God.

7. God is Sovereign over all things and rules over all kingdoms:

"For the Lord of hosts has purposed, and who will annul it? His hand is stretched out, and who will turn it back?" (Isaiah 14:27 ESV)

God is unstoppable! No one can successful oppose Him. With Him on your side, your victory is guaranteed.

"And said, O Lord, God of our fathers, are You not God in heaven? And do You not rule over all the kingdoms of the nations? In Your hand are power and might, so that none is able to withstand You" (2 Chronicles 20:6 AMP).

God is your sure connection. One with God is majority.

8. God is infinitely wise:

"Oh, how great are God's riches and wisdom and knowledge! How impossible it is for us to understand his decisions and his ways!" (Romans 11:33 NLT)

Another reason why you should trust God to keep His Word is that He is infinitely wise. He knows what you do not know. He sees far beyond what you are seeing. He sees the end from the very beginning and knows what is perfect for you.

9. God has wonderful plans for you:

"For I know the plans I have for you," says the Lord. "They are plans for good and not for disaster, to give you a future and a hope" (Jeremiah 29:11 NLT).

You can be rest assured that your plans are nothing compared to the plans God have for you. No one knows you like your maker. He knows why He created you and knows exactly what suits you. You cannot live a fruitful and fulfilling life without His help.

10. God loves and cares for you:

God loves you unconditionally. Even if you were the only one on earth, do you know God would have still sent Jesus to die for just you? Your worth to God is the life of Jesus. He loves you so much and that is why He craves for your fellowship.

"But God showed his great love for us by sending Christ to die for us while we were still sinners" (Romans 5:8 NLT).

God is concerned about every single thing that concerns you even to the smallest detail. Not even a strand of your hair falls to the ground without His notice.

"Casting the whole of your care [all your anxieties, all your worries, all your concerns, once and for all] on Him, for He cares for you affectionately and cares about you watchfully" (1 Peter 5:7 AMP).

God wants you healed, His will for you is that you live in perfect health, but you have to trust Him and act on His word through faith.

How to Build Your Faith for Divine Healing

"So then faith cometh by hearing, and hearing by the word of God" (Romans 10:17). Faith for divine healing comes by hearing God's word on divine healing repeatedly. To build your faith for divine healing, you must personalize and confess God's word on healing until the truth of God's word on healing comes alive in your heart (spirit).

Unless the word of God for healing moves from your head (mind) to your heart, you will struggle to receive healing. That is why you must meditate on what God's word says about healing. The more you meditate, the more you build up faith, until you become strong enough in the faith to take your healing out of the spirit realm into the natural realm of sense, and your healing will appear for all to see.

Whether or not you receive your healing, healing is your covenant right. It is a matter of choice. That is why God said, "I have given you the choice between life and death, between blessings and curses. Now I call on heaven and earth to witness the choice you make. Oh, that you would choose life, so that you and your descendants might live!" (Deuteronomy 30:19 NLT).

Here are scriptures that will enable you to build your faith so you can receive divine healing from God.

<u>Scriptures to Build Your Faith for Divine Healing</u>
1. Healing is God's will for All:

Jesus healed ALL the sick that came to Him for healing in Matthew 8:16. There is not an instance He turned down anyone who came to Him for healing. The Bible chronicles seventeen instances Jesus healed ALL the sick that were presence. Every one of them got healed.

You can read about those instances in Matthew 4:22-24; 18:16-19; 9:35; 12:15; 14:14; 14:34-36; 15:30-31; 19:2; 21:14; Mark 1:32-34; 1:39; 6:56; Luke 4:40; 6:17-19; 7:21; 9:11 and 17:12-17. At other times, Jesus healed one or two people who needed healing, and you will find 47 of such occasion. But not for once did He refuse anyone healing. And He certainly will not turn you down.

Healing is God's will for ALL. The fact that Jesus healed ALL attest to this truth because we know He never did anything outside of God's will. "Then answered Jesus and said unto them, Verily, verily, I say unto you, The Son can do nothing of himself, but what he seeth the Father do: for what things soever he doeth, these also doeth the Son likewise" (John 5:19).

2. Healing is God's will for you:

God wants you well, that is why He said, "Beloved, I wish above all things that thou mayest prosper and be in health, even as thy soul prospereth" (3 John 1:2). Healing is God's will and there is absolutely no sickness or disease He cannot heal. "Bless the LORD, O my soul, and forget not all his benefits: Who forgiveth all thine iniquities; who healeth all thy diseases" (Psalms 103:2-3).

3. God already sent Jesus for your healing:

God is not going to send Jesus to heal you, He already did. One of the reasons Jesus came was so you will be healed. He came and settled everything that concerns your healing. Your healing is a done deal. It is now your responsibility to take your healing. The Bible tells us in John 1:1, 14 that Jesus is the word of God made flesh. God already sent His Word (Jesus) to heal you. "He sent his word, and healed them, and delivered them from their destructions" (Psalms 107:20).

4. Sickness is a curse and you have been redeemed from it:

When you read the book of Deuteronomy 28: 15-68, you will notice that God referred to sicknesses and diseases as curse. The good news however, is that Jesus Christ has redeemed us from every curse, including sickness and disease now present and those to be discovered. "Christ hath redeemed us from the curse of the law, being made a curse for us: for it is written, Cursed is every one that hangeth on a tree" (Galatians 3;13).

5. Your healing is a done deal:

Healing is in Christ's Atonement. Jesus paid for your healing when He paid for your sins. "But he was wounded for our transgressions, he was bruised for our iniquities: the chastisement of our peace was upon him; and with his stripes we are healed" (Isaiah 53:5).

"This was to fulfil what was spoken by the prophet Isaiah: He took our illness and bore our diseases" (Matthew 8:17 NLT).

"Who his own self bare our sins in his own body on the tree, that we, being dead to sins, should live unto righteousness: by whose stripes ye were healed" (1 Peter 2:24).

The stripes Jesus received on His back were specifically for your healing. The truth is that Jesus has already healed you, it is now a matter of receiving what is now yours legally. In Christ Jesus, healing is our covenant right. You must know who you are and what is yours so you won't be cheated out of what is rightly yours. You must be Christ conscious!

In key #4: D for "Don't be casual with illness, exercise your dominion", our focus will be on how to receive healing. By now, I am sure you already know it is going to be by faith. So be wise enough to read and meditate on the scriptures on healing until you build up the faith to receive your healing. The moment the Word of God on healing comes alive in your spirit, your healing will manifest.

Now the just shall live by faith: but if any man draw back, my soul shall have no pleasure in him" (Hebrews 10:38); because without faith it is impossible to please God (Hebrews 11:6).

KEY #3: C - CONSCIOUSNESS: KNOW WHO YOU ARE

"Your identity is your most valuable possession. Protect It." - Elastigirl from The Incredible.
"A man who stands for nothing will fall for anything" - Malcolm X.

I know you are you, but how exactly is "you" defined? If I ask "who are you?" you will most probably answer by telling me your name, family background, educational qualifications, job and hobbies. Are those really your true identity?

Your identity is your inner you, your core, if you like, it is your operating software. It is not what you do and why you do what you do. It goes far beyond that. You are much more than your job, gender, race or what has happened to your or even what you are going through right now. So, who exactly are you?

Who are you?

The only person with the accurate understanding of a product is the manufacturer. You cannot claim to know a product better than the manufacturer(s). Most products come with operational manual from the manufacturer(s) detailing how to use the products. Only the manufacturer of a product can tell you the right way to use the product because no one understands the product like the maker. Without manufacturer's instruction on how best to use a product, abuse will set in.

We are God's products, and He created every one of us unique for a purpose. To fully understand who you are, you must turn to your maker, the Almighty God. He is the only One who can tell you exactly who you are. And until you know who you are and your purpose, purposeful and fulfilling life becomes an illusion.

The beginning of awareness is the embrace of God's invitation for friendship made possible through Jesus Christ. Through fellowship with God, your soul is connected to His fountain of wisdom and knowledge. Then you begin to see yourself as God sees you. You are who God says you are and you can do exactly what He says you can do.

The Lost Identity

Man lost his identity when his core became corrupted. Man's operating system crashed completely when in the Garden of Eden, man chose to obey Satan and committed high treason against His maker. Man fell from grace, and sin like virus corrupted man's essence.

The fall of our first parents, Adam and Eve, brought the entire natural world and mankind into Satan's dominion. Every man born into this world is therefore born into original sin, like a software installed in a virus-infected computer. Man lost touch with God and soon started to malfunction.

Man lost his identity because he lost touch with his maker. And until man reconnect to God, he will remain a shadow of himself. True meaning of life is found in God and God alone. An unregenerate man cannot fellowship with God. God is a spirit, to fellowship with Him, you must be born of the Spirit (John 4:24).

Meet your true self

The death and resurrection of Jesus Christ has made it possible for us to be set free from Satan's dominion and be adopted into God's kingdom as His children. To be translated to God's kingdom, you must first be born again, and become a new creature.

"This means that anyone who belongs to Christ has become a new person. The old life is gone; a new life has begun!" (2 Corinthians 5:17) "For He has rescued us from the kingdom of darkness and transferred us into the kingdom of His dear Son." (Colossians 1:13 NLT)

Every born again child of God has a new identity and reality in Christ. Accept your new identity and walk in agreement with God. See yourself through God's eyes and carry yourself in that image.

Many who are victims of life are actually victims of ignorance and not to devil. "My people are destroyed for lack of knowledge..." He didn't say my people are destroyed because of the devil, He said ignorance is the destroyer. God said in Psalms 82:6 that, "you are gods, sons of the Most High", but because you are ignorant of who you are (Psalms 82:5), you will die like mere men (Psalms 82:7).

Your life is based on the information you have about

who you are. Think about it, how would you live if you realize that no sickness or disease can afflict your body? The quality of your life is directly related to your level of knowledge.

"And wisdom and knowledge shall be the stability of thy times, and strength of salvation: the fear of the LORD is his treasure" (Isaiah 33:6).

Your life will turn out great if you fill your heart with the knowledge of God's word. Through meditating on the Word of God, you get to learn who you are and what you are capable of. The Word of God, the Bible, is God's manual for daily living. It is your identity manual. It is a mirror that reflects your true identity.

"And all of us, as with unveiled face, [because we] continued to behold [in the Word of God] as in a mirror the glory of the Lord, are constantly being transfigured into His very own image in ever increasing splendour and from one degree of glory to another; [for this comes] from the Lord [Who is] the Spirit" (2 Corinthians 3:18).

Christ Consciousness

"For [as far as this world is concerned] you have died, and your [new, real] life is hidden with Christ in God" (Colossians 3:3).

When the reality of your true identity in Christ dawns on you, you suddenly realize that you have dominion over life challenges. Your Christ consciousness will put you over the world and you will realize that the world does not determine what happens to you.

In Christ Jesus, we have eternal life, the very life of God. This life makes you live above sickness, disease, defeat and everything that is of darkness.

You must confess who you are in Christ. For example, when you hear a Christian say, "I am sick" or "I am diabetic" or "I have cancer", you know immediately that that fellow does not know who he or she is in Christ Jesus. Imagine a Christian claiming sickness when the Bible says, "No one in Zion will say, "I'm sick" (Isaiah 33:24 MSG). Such a Christian have not developed the Christ-consciousness.

You are a god, a child of the Most High God, the God of gods, you have been born into Zion, a place of absolute health (Isaiah 33:24, Hebrews 12: 22 - 24). You have the very life of God flowing in you, because you have been made a partaker of God's divine nature (2 Peter 1:4). Your human life that was susceptible to sickness and disease has been supplanted by the life of God.

KEY #4: D - DON'T BE CASUAL WITH ILLNESS, EXERCISE YOUR DOMINION

"Rise up, set out on your journey and go over the valley of the Arnon. Behold, I have given into your hand Sihon the Amorite, king of Heshbon, and his land. Begin to take possession, and contend with him in battle" (Deuteronomy 2:24 ESV).

The Lord told the children of Israel He had given into their hands the king of Hishbon and his land, but they have to possess it through contention (battle). The promises of God are not fulfilled automatically. There is always something to be done to appropriate God's promises into your life. Though God had given the children of Israel the land of the king of Heshbon, if they do nothing to possess it, they won't have it and God will not force them to contend for it.

God Will Not Override Your Authority

God gave us free will. It means we can choose to accept or reject God. We can choose to obey or disobey His instructions, but for every action we take, there are consequences, whether good or bad.

God gave Adam authority and he chose to relinquish it to the devil, and God did not override his decision. God has given you and I authority and dominion in Christ Jesus and He won't override our authority.

God will let you die in sin and go to hell if you choose to do so. God will let you die sick too if you chose to. It is up to you to accept Jesus and His gift of righteousness. It is equally up to you to believe and accept the healing scriptures in the Bible and all that God has made available to you in Christ Jesus. The choice is yours and God will not stop you, however, with every choice, there are consequences.

The Bible makes it clear that you have been healed already. You can choose to believe God and receive your healing or keep crying and begging Him to heal you. In Isaiah 53:5, the Bible said, "But he was wounded for our transgressions, he was bruised for our iniquities: the chastisement of our peace was upon him; and with his stripes we are healed". Notice the past tense "healed" signifying that it's done. The Bible did not say "by His stripe we will be healed", it said "we are healed". It up to you to believe God and His Word.

The fact that the Bible said Jesus has healed you already by His stripes does not mean you will experience healing automatically. The children of Israel had to contend with the king of Heshbon before they could possess the land God had given them. Healing is yours but the devil won't let you have it. You have to contend with him to receive your healing. You have to fight a good fight of faith (1 Timothy 6:12). It must be by faith, and it is called the "good fight" because your victory is guaranteed.

"For whatsoever is born of God overcometh the world: and this is the victory that overcometh the world, even our faith" (1 John 5:4).

God has given you dominion over all powers of the enemy (Satan), exercise your dominion to get what you want through faith (Luke 10:19).

You receive your healing the exact same way you receive salvation. God tells us how to receive salvation in Romans 10: 9-10,

"That if thou shalt confess with thy mouth the Lord Jesus, and shalt believe in thine heart that God hath raised him from the dead, thou shalt be saved. For with the heart man believeth unto righteousness; and with the mouth confession is made unto salvation".

To receive your healing, you must first acknowledge that healing is God's will for you. You must believe in your heart with no iota of doubt that Jesus healed you over 2,000 years ago when He received those stripes on His back (1 Peter 2:24). Finally, you must receive your healing by confessing it is yours through faith.

"We having the same spirit of faith, according as it is written, I believed, and therefore have I spoken; we also believe, and therefore speak" (2 Corinthians 4:13).

It is not enough to believe, you must confess what you believe.

Taking Responsibility

Some people are so casual with illness as though it is normal to be ill. Others take illness so lightly until it gets serious and they start running from pillar to post. Sickness is curse and there is nothing normal about curses. Every sickness no matter how minor it seems is an agent of death. Sickness and Satan share common mission: "To steal, and to kill, and to destroy" (John 10:10).

Until you vehemently resist and oppose sickness, it will remain.

"From the days of John the Baptist until now the kingdom of heaven has suffered violence, and the violent take it by force" (John 11:12 ESV).

Do you want healing? It's yours already, but you must take is by force. You don't pray for it, you take it. You have to "fight the good fight of faith" to lay hold on it (1 Timothy 6:120.

God wants you well and to walk in divine health, that is why He sent Jesus to pay for your healing. Healing is in Christ's Atonement - by "His stripes" you are healed! God has done everything He needs to do for your healing; you must take responsibility for your healing.

Stop acting as if God made you sick or does not want you healed. The enemy here is not God but Satan. You must take sides with God against your common enemy - the devil.

Why not just stop crying and begging God for what He has already made available for you. Take responsibility. Do what He asked you to do, resist the devil and the sickness he brought and he will flee from you (James 4:7).

There are Christians who erroneously believe God made them sick to teach them something. How can God after sending Jesus to pay for your healing put sickness on you. It is like saying God is the reason why you commit sin.

How can the God who sent Jesus to die for your sin make you commit sin, does that make sense? God does not and will never use sickness to teach us anything, He uses His Word and the Holy Spirit. God wants you healed. He wants you to live in divine health. He said,

"Beloved, I wish above all things that thou mayest prosper and be in health, even as thy soul prospereth" (3 John 1:2).

The more knowledge you have about God love, the easier it becomes to receive your healing. God loves you so much that He does not want you ill. No sane parent will want his or her child sick or remain sick, how much more our loving heavenly Father.

"He that spared not his own Son, but delivered him up for us all, how shall he not with him also freely give us all things?" (Romans 8:32).

Some of the things God has given us to freely enjoy are salvation, healing and divine health.

Healing is yours, take it. In Christ Jesus, we are healed. We are not the sick trying to get healed. We are the healed the devil is trying put sickness on. We must not allow him.

<u>Exercising your Dominion in Christ is Obedience not Pride</u>

"Behold, I give unto you power to tread on serpents and scorpions, and over all the power of the enemy: and nothing shall by any means hurt you" (Luke 10:19).

Jesus gave us authority but it is up to us to use it. If you desire to receive healing, then you must use your God given authority in Christ Jesus.

Some Christians and even church leaders feel it is better to pray to God for healing and not to command healing in the name of Jesus. They think it is pride when you exercise your God given authority in Christ Jesus to command sickness to leave your body or the body of others. They is no humility is praying for what is yours already, it is ignorance. Neither is it pride to exercise your authority over the devil and everything that he brought, as a matter of fact, it is obedience to God.

In Acts 3:6-8, Peter certainly didn't pray to God to heal the cripple man at the beautiful gate, he commanded the lame man to walk in Jesus' Name. In Acts 16:18, Paul delivered a certain damsel possessed of the spirit of divination not by praying but by commanding the fowl spirit in the Name of Jesus. In Acts 9:34, Peter healed a man that was bed-ridden for eight years. He simply said, "Aeneas, Jesus Christ maketh thee whole: Arise, and make thy bed" and the man got up immediately, completely healed.

Healing is yours, Jesus has healed you over 2,000 years ago by His stripes and He has given you authority to tread upon Satan and everything that represents him. Exercise your authority today! Stop talking about sickness and disease and rebuke them. We were not ask to talk about the mountain but to cast them out (Mark 11:23). Your body is the temple of the Holy Spirit, don't accommodate sickness in it. Command that sickness and all the symptoms of sickness in your body to leave in the name of Jesus.

When you take authority over your body, say, "I receive healing in Jesus Name. I rebuke every symptom in my body right now, in Jesus' Name. I am healed from the crown of my head to the sole of my feet in the name of Jesus. I take my healing! I am healed! Glory to God! Hallelujah!"

KEY #5: E – EXPECT HEALING MANIFESTATION

"I tell you the truth, you can say to this mountain, 'May you be lifted up and thrown into the sea', and it will happen. But you must really believe it will happen and have no doubt in your heart. I tell you, you can pray for anything, and if you believe that you've received it, it will be yours" (Mark 11:23-24).

To receive your healing, you must first believe that it is yours in Christ Jesus. The Bible says you have been healed by His stripes (Isaiah 53:5). It is not enough to believe, you must receive it by faith and confess it is yours. But it doesn't stop there, you must look forward to seeing the manifestation.

Faith does not stop at believing and confessing, you must really anticipate for what you hope for. You must be hundred percent persuaded that what you hope for must come to pass. You are healed the moment you received your healing by faith. You receive healing spiritually and you walk in divine health by faith. When you receive healing, it may manifest instantly or it may be gradual, so in case its taking time to manifest, don't let the lingering symptoms cause you to doubt.

Nothing aborts miracle like doubt. Don't give room to

doubt if you want to see the manifestation of your healing. Cast out every thought and imagination that devil sends your way.

You have got to learn to walk by faith and not by sight. Remember that when we got saved, nothing happened on the outside, but nevertheless we became an entirely new creature (2 Corinthians 5:17). It took some time for people to begin to notice that something has happened in and to us. That is how it is with divine healing, if you believed you are healed, then you are, symptoms notwithstanding.

If you don't believe your healing until you see it, you won't receive it from God. Believing precedes receiving. You must stand on God's word until your healing manifest for all to see to the glory of God. When the manifestation of your healing lingers, know that God is waiting on you to stand against the devil and bring it into being. So, don't stop confessing it is yours, don't stop thanking God for it and don't stop rebuking every lying symptoms of the devil until they disappear.

As good as divine healing is, divine health is better. So, even after the manifestation of your healing, don't stop confessing that divine health is yours in Christ Jesus. Keep confessing that by the stripe of Jesus you are healed and live and walk day-to-day in divine health. Confess that total and perfect health is yours in Christ Jesus. Remember that the power of life and death is in your mouth and you can always have what you say. Use your mouth to stay healthy.

KEY #6: F – FOLLOWING IN THE STEPS OF FATHER ABRAHAM

"Look unto Abraham your father, and unto Sarah that bare you: for I called him alone, and blessed him, and increased him" (Isaiah 51:2).

No sermon on faith is perfectly complete that does not make reference to the father of faith, Abraham. Even God has asked us to look unto him. God wants us to follow in his steps. Abraham, the founder of the Hebrews nation, became the 'friend of God' through his faith and obedience. Abraham believed whatever God said. He was driven by the belief that if God promised something, God has the integrity, ability and desire to bring it to pass. His faith was based on God's character and nature.

God promised Abraham and Serah a son, through whom He will bless and make Abraham a father of many nations. Though Abraham and Serah were already old and Serah was barren, yet he believed God. He believed that God was able to do what He promised.

In Romans 4:18, the Bibles tells us how Abraham believed in hope in hopeless situation and refused to stagger at the promise of God through unbelief. He was fully persuaded that God was able to bring His promise to pass, it was inputted unto him for righteousness.

Are you in a hopeless situation right now? Have you been told that your illness is terminal? It is up to you whether to believe the report of man or that of God. You have got to find out for yourself what God says concerning your health. Only God has the final say.

The Bible says in Matthew 8:17, "Himself took our infirmities, and bare our sicknesses" The Word makes it clear that Jesus already took away your illness. If He took it away, it means you don't have it anymore. All you have to do is believe God. God is not a liar, He says whatever He means and means every single Word He says. If He said you are healed, then you are, how you feel and what the doctors have said notwithstanding.

Like Abraham, you have got to be fully persuaded that God's Word is absolutely true. By the stripes of Jesus, you have been healed and that is final. All you need do is believe and thankfully receive your healing by confessing you are healed.

"He staggered not at the promise of God through unbelief, but was strong in faith, giving glory to God" (Romans 4:20).

Long before Isaac came, Abraham kept thanking God for him. Though it was naturally impossible for him and Serah to birth a child, yet he had an unshakable faith God will make the impossible possible. You too have to believe God for your healing manifestation irrespective of how you feel or what the doctors have said.

Strong faith gives glory to God for what is yet to be, while weak faith grumbles for what isn't manifested. Any time you start lamenting about your condition, faith is not in place. Faith lives from the invisible towards the visible. Faith lives from the spiritual to the natural real of perception.

You receive divine healing by faith, and by faith you walk and live day-to-day in divine health. Faith comes by repeatedly hearing the Word of God. Keep confessing God's Word on health. Declare to yourself aloud that you are healed. Declare that the symptoms are disappearing and that you walk and live in divine health.

Remember that faith is fixing your attention on the unseen realm of the spirit. Unbelief is focusing on what you can perceive with your natural sense organs. Take your mind off symptoms and pain and fasten it on God's Word. That is how to follow in the steps of father, Abraham.

KEY #7: G – GIVING REVERENCE TO GOD

Giving reverence to God means to acknowledge God's Lordship over your life. It means to have deep respect for His person and to obey what He commands.

Reverence of God also means to fear Him and to honor His Name. Reverence or fear of God starts from the heart and manifests in our actions and words. It is not an outward things but the inward disposition of the heart towards God which permeates to the outside.

The Almighty God has promised divine healing for all that fear His Name.

"But unto you that fear my name shall the Sun of righteousness arise with healing in his wings..." (Malachi 4:2).

Are you interested in living in divine health? One of the keys to living in divine health is to fear the Lord, to acknowledge His Lordship and obey His commandments.

Jesus is the Sun of righteousness and healing is in His wings. The fear of God means giving Jesus the first place in your life. When you diligently obey the Word of God, sickness and diseases will be far from you.

God is Holy and to be at right standing with Him, you

must pursue holiness (1 Peter 1:15-16). You must say no to every form of ungodliness and worldly passions. The fear of God calls for self-control and departure from every appearance of sin (Titus 2:12).

Giving reverence to God also means to constantly worship God. The only thing God craves for is Worship. And the natural response to heart that is transformed by the Holy Spirit is that of worship and reverence because we were created to fellowship and worship God. God has invited us to intimate walk with Him but you must be very careful not to allow familiarity with God breed contempt, but greater reverence.

Let me reemphasize that reverence for God is not an outward show, but our inward disposition to God. God looks at the heart. And as long as your heart is right with Him, He is committed to seeing that no plague comes near you or your dwelling.

Here are ten ways to practice reverence

1. Treasure God's name

2. Live a holy and blameless life

3. Treat yourself and others respectfully

4. Love God with all your heart

5. Praise God always joyfully

6. Exalt the Lord above anyone, everything and anything

7. Desire to know Him more

8. Love what He loves and have whatever He hates

9. Trust and believe God and His Word and be willing to do anything He ask of you with joy

10. Approach Him with great humility and acknowledge Him as the greatest.

When you practice the above, you will live your life in divine health because God said so (Malachi 4:2).

KEY #8: H – HEALING POWER OF THE HOLY GHOST

The Holy Ghost is the healer and the giver of the healing power. One of the gifts of the Holy Spirit is the gift of healing.

"To another faith by the same Spirit; to another the gifts of healing by the same Spirit" (1 Corinthians 12:9).

The Holy Spirit was the one behind every single healing miracle Jesus performed while He walked the earth. The Bible confirms this in Acts 10:38, where it says,

"How God anointed Jesus of Nazareth with the Holy Ghost and with power: who went about doing good, and healing all that were oppressed of the devil; for God was with him".

The good news is that the Holy Spirit, the great healer lives with us and in us today. Hallelujah!

"And I will pray the Father, and He shall give you another Comforter, that He may abide with you for ever; even the Spirit of truth; whom the world cannot receive, because it seeth Him not, neither knoweth Him: but ye know Him; for He dwelleth with you, and shall be in you" (John 14: 15 – 16).

The Holy Spirit came to earth to stay on the day of Pentecost. He will be with us to the end of time. Unlike Jesus who could be only in one place at a time when He walked the earth, the Holy Spirit can be everywhere, all the time, and He reside in those who have accepted Jesus Christ as their Lord and Savior.

When you give your life to Jesus, you are born again, born of the Spirit and your body becomes the abode of the Holy Spirit. Now imagine the Healer, the one who gives the gift of healing, the one behind all the healing miracles of Jesus, imagine Him dwelling inside of you. With Him in you, how can you be sick? He will give life to your body. If you are filled with the Holy Ghost and you are not living in divine health, you are simple ignorant of who you carry.

"But if the Spirit of Him who raised Jesus from the dead dwells in you, He who raised Christ Jesus from the dead will also give life to your mortal bodies through His Spirit who dwells in you" (Romans 8:11).

Your body is the temple of the Holy Spirit, not sickness. Do not accommodate sickness in your body. Use your mouth to keep sickness far from you. How intimate is your fellowship with the Holy Spirit? You have got to be conscious of who you carry. That way He will bring healing and restoration to your soul: your mind, will and emotions.

Through the Holy Spirit, you can live in divine health – spirit, soul and body. He wants you to live in divine health, so you will have the vitality to fulfill God's mandate for your life. God wants you to live in divine health and never to need healing. You are to bring healing to others. That is why He gives the gift of healing. And has asked us to pray and lay hands on the sick. You can't lay hand on the sick when you yourself is sick. You have got to walk in divine health, and the key is the indwelling presence of the Holy Spirit.

By the grace of God, I have walked and lived in divine

health for about fourteen years now (since 2006), and I will continue to live in divine health all my life. It is not by my power or might, but by the power of the Holy Spirit (Zechariah 4:6). Today, I am extending the Healing power of the Holy Ghost to others through my blog posts, books and messages. You too can walk in divine health and become a channel through which others can receive their healing.

Do you have the Holy Spirit residing inside of you? To be baptized in the Holy Ghost, you must be born again. Perhaps you are not born again, this is your moment. Open your hear to Jesus and receive Him as your Lord and Savior.

To receive the baptism of the Holy Spirit, pray the prayer below:

<u>Prayer for Baptism in the Holy Spirit</u>

Heaven Father, You said in your word, "If ye then, being evil, know how to give good gifts unto your children: how much more shall your heavenly Father GIVE THE HOLY SPIRIT to them that ASK Him?" (Luke 11:13). With faith in your word, I ask that You fill me with the Holy Spirit.

Holy Spirit, I welcome You, rise up within me as I praise God. Give me utterance to speak with other tongues (Acts 2:4). In Jesus' Name. Amen.

Remember, one of the keys to living in divine health is the indwelling presence of the Holy Spirit. Make it a habit to fellowship with the Holy Spirit all the time.

The Holy Spirit is a person, equal with the Father and the Son. You can't be filled with the Holy Spirit and harbor sickness in your body, never!

KEY #9: I – INCLINE YOUR EARS TO MY SAYING

The word of God is

"life to those who find them, healing and health to all their flesh"
(Proverbs 4:22 AMP).

Do you need healing? Or perhaps, you want to go beyond healing to living a divine health. The secret is to fix your undivided attention on God's word.

Sickness of any kind distracts. The devil uses sickness and diseases to keep us focus on pain and discomfort, and distracted from the word of God. He knows that he cannot make you ill or keep you in ailment when you constantly meditate on the word of life, paying attention and listening to every instruction of God for an extraordinary life of victory.

One of the keys to living in divine health is to always incline your ears to God's word. To incline your ears means to actively and carefully consider. It can be likened to a man leaning forward, tipping his head to hear more clearly, so he can listen to pay attention to details.

To incline your ears to God's word means to shut out everything around you, and, without any distraction and interruptions, give your undivided attention to His word. That is how to attend to His word. When you do, His word will produce life, healing and health to all your flesh.

"My son, attend to my words; incline thine ear unto my sayings. Let them not depart from thine eyes; keep them in the midst of thine heart. For they are life unto those that find them, and health to all their flesh" (Proverbs 4: 20 – 22).

You have to be careful what you constantly listen to. In Mark 4:24, Jesus cautioned us to pay attention to what we hear. Why? Because you become what you hear. What you constantly hear forms your thought, and a man becomes what he constantly think about. This is because you speak out of the abundance of your heart, and the power of life and death is in your tongue. So, from the abundance of your heart, you either speak life or death, sickness or health, poverty or prosperity, defeat or victory, faith or fear, etc.

Faith comes by hearing and hearing by the word of God. Fear, defeat, sickness and death comes by hearing and hearing the lies of the devil. You have to pay attention to what you allow into your heart. You have to think about what you constantly think about. The proof that you are paying enough attention to God's word is that His word becomes your word and His word becomes the motive for your actions.

Do you want to live a sickness free life? Feed your heart with the life giving word of God. "The words that I speak unto you, they are spirit, and they are life (John 6:63). The word of God is a seed that produces life (salvation, health and prosperity). You can't be filled with God's word and not live in divine health. The word of God is full of power too great to comprehend. And the Word produces what it promises.

The Bible tells us, in Psalms 107:20, that God sent His Word and the Word healed the sick and delivered the oppressed from destructions. It means that no sickness or destruction can come near you if you are loaded with the Word.

I pray for you today, as you begin to incline your ears to the word of God, to pay attention to His sayings, you are released from all discomforts and sickness, and your health is restored, in Jesus' Name. Amen.

KEY #10: J – JOYFUL HEART

Proverbs 17:22 (MSG) says, "A joyful heart is good medicine, but a broken spirit dries up the bone".

You are either joyful or gloomy (having a broken spirit). While a joyful, happy, cheerful disposition is good for your health, a broken spirit on the other hand leads to anxiety, depression and spiritual and physical drainage. A broken spirit leads to feeling of hopelessness and lack of strength to persevere.

One of the keys to living in divine health is to have a joyful heart. The word "heart" as used by the Bible refers to our spirit man or inner man or our true self. It is your responsibility to ensure you stay joyful or cheerful even when life is stressful and hard. Happiness comes from within, not without. If you are waiting for others to make you happy, you may never be happy. It is up to you if you will be joyful or not.

It is important to note also that "joyful" heart does not mean smiling and laughing all the time. It does not mean jumping up and down grinning from ear to ear. It goes beyond that. Joyfulness is an inward disposition which is seen through outward expression of smiles or our heart. You can smile and not be joyful, but you can't be joyful and not be full of smiles.

"A joyful heart makes a cheerful face, but when the heart is sad, the spirit is broken" (Proverbs 15:13 NASB).

Do you want to live in divine health? Do you want sickness to be far from you? Pay attention to your heart. Fix your thought on things that promote a joyful heart. The Bible tells us what to think about in Philippians 4:8, "And now, dear brothers and sisters, one final thing. Fix your thoughts on what is true, and honorable, and right, and pure, and lovely, and admirable. Think about things that are excellent and worthy of praise".

Did you know that happy people tend to live longer and experience better health than unhappy people? Feeling positive about yourself and life contributes to both better health and longevity. Why not make up your mind to live happy irrespective of the circumstances you find yourself. Avoid stress, anxiety and depressing thoughts. Do not wait for others to make you happy, take responsibility for your happiness.

There is no denying the fact that our emotional health is connected to our physical health. Those who have a joyful and positive outlook undeniably have better physical health. But the question is, "how can one maintain a joyful heart when life throw things on us that will steal away our joy and peace?" So, here are few ways to keep the joy deep within us.

1. His Presence:
Spending quality time in God's presence guarantees a

joyful heart.

> *"Thou wilt shew me the path of life: in thy presence is fullness of joy: at thy right hand there are pleasures for evermore" (Psalms 16:11).*

2. Have an attitude of gratitude:

If you want a tank full of joy and peace, be thankful.

> *"Don't worry about anything; instead, pray about everything. Tell God what you need, and thank Him for all He has done. Then you will experience God's peace, which exceeds anything we can understand. His peace will guard your hearts and minds as you live in Christ Jesus" (Philippians 4: 6 – 7 NLT).*

3. Answered Prayer:

Nothing brings joy like answered prayer. That is why you have to learn to pray according to God's will. God answers all prayers prayed according to His will.

> *"Ask, and you will receive, that your joy may be full" (John 16:24 ESV).*

4. Meditate on God's Word:

The word of God brings joy. Spend quality time meditating on the word of God.

> *"These things have I spoken unto you, that my joy might remain in you, and that your joy might be full" (John 15:11).*

5. Fellowship of saints:

There is great joy when we gather in fellowship as one family.

> *"Greatly desiring to see thee... that I may be filled with joy" (2 Timothy 1:4).*

Now you know that keeping your joy, is one of the keys to living in divine health. Decide that you will have a joyful heart every day, circumstances notwithstanding.

May the joy of the Lord keep you in perfect peace and health in Jesus' Name (Amen).

KEY #11: K – KINGDOM SERVICE

Kingdom Service is the eleventh of the 26 keys to living in divine health. No employer will want his or her valuable employee, who contributes greatly to the growth of the company to be sick. That is why most companies have medical allowance because they want their employees healthy. How much more God?

God does not want to lose anyone who is actively involved in His kingdom service to sickness. As a stakeholder in God's kingdom, your service is highly needed, and God is committed to seeing that you live in divine health.

Kingdom service is one of the keys to living in divine health. In the Book of Exodus, God promised to keep sickness far from those who serve Him faithfully.

"And ye shall serve the Lord your God, and he shall bless thy bread, and thy water; and I will take sickness away from the midst of thee" (Exodus 23:25).

Do you want to live in total and perfect health? Serve God with all your heart, with all your soul and with all your mind. Serve Him wholeheartedly. You have got to put God's agenda first in your life, when you do, all things, including divine health will be added unto you (Matthew 6:33).

There is great reward in serving and pleasing God. One of the rewards is that you will never grow weary and your vitality is renewed daily and you will be strengthened to fulfill your life assignment.

Make up your mind today to become useful to God, to submit to Him in total humility, and be actively involved in advancing His course here on earth. Join a local Church and be committed, and whatsoever you do, do it heartily, as to the Lord, and not unto men.

KEY #12: L – LEAN ON GOD

Man is a spirit with soul living in a body. God gave us our bodies as gift, and He has made available the owner's manual, the Bible, which contains instructions we need to take care of our bodies.

In the Bible, you will discover instructions on how to take good care of yourself so that you can live long and live in divine health. One of the keys to living in divine health in the scripture that people hardly think of is found in Proverbs 3: 5 - 8, where the Bible makes it clear that trusting God is good for your health.

Why is trusting and leaning on God good for your health? God has promised all those who put their trust in Him peace. When you lean on God, God's peace that surpasses all understanding will guard your heart. And "a peaceful heart leads to a healthy body" (Proverbs 14:30 NLT).

When it comes to living in health, what you eat is very important, but most important is what eats you. You cannot live in divine health when you are filled with worry, fear, bitterness, resentment, or any other emotional disease.

The good news is that we can overcome every form of emotional disease simply by trusting God and leaning totally on Him. Trusting God is one of the keys to living in divine health that cannot fail. So, how do we trust in God? Proverbs 3: 5 – 11 tells us how. We will quickly look at the passage.

"Trust in the Lord with all your heart and do not lean on your own understanding. In all your ways acknowledge Him and He will make your paths straight. Do not be wise in your own eyes; Fear the Lord and turn away from evil. It will be healing to your body and refreshment to your bones" (Proverbs 3: 5 – 8 NASB).

Here are the steps to follow to make sure you are trusting and leaning on the Lord.

1. Don't lean on your own understanding, but depend totally on God. Proverbs 3:5.

2. Surrender totally to God in your thoughts, words and actions. Proverbs 3:6.

3. Shun evil and flee every appearance of sin. Stay clear from anything and everyone that can hinder your relationship with God. Proverbs 3:7.

4. Put God first in your life. Don't let anything and anyone come before God in your life. Proverbs 3: 9 - 10.

5. X-Ray your life with God's word and jettison whatever that is not of God in your life. Proverbs 3:11.

When you follow the steps above, "it will be healing to your body and refreshing to your bones" (Proverbs 3:8).

KEY #13: M – MAINTAIN THE RIGHT ENVIRONMENT

Your body is your first environment. You are a spirit being with a soul living in an environment called body. Your body is also an abode of the Spirit of God. You glorify God when you take proper care of your body and live a healthy lifestyle.

Your body has been purchased by God, hence God will hold you responsible if your abuse your body. God built a mechanism called immune system that helps the body fight sicknesses and diseases. It is your responsibility to take care of your body so as to not weaken your body's immune system.

"Or do you not know that your body is a temple of the Holy Spirit within you, whom you have from God? You are not your own, for you were bought with a price. So, glorify God in your body (1 Corinthians 6: 19 – 20).

Apart from your body, where you dwell is also your environment. The earth is the Lord's but He has entrusted its care to us. It is our responsibility to cultivate, guard and use the earth wisely if we must live in total and perfect health.

"The heavens belong to the Lord, but He has given the earth to all humanity" (Psalms 115:16 NLT).

Carelessness on the part of man to maintain clean and

hygiene environment accounts for most of the sicknesses and diseases that plague man today. God wants us to live long and be in health (3 John 1:2), so He gave man specific directions for hygiene and cleanliness.

In Deuteronomy 23: 12 – 14, God gave the children of Israel guidelines for hygiene and sanitation, so they can enjoy good health and be protected against sickness and diseases.

Do you want to live in health? Keep your surrounding clean. You need safe, sanitary and peaceful environment to live in divine health.

Another environment to pay attention to if we must walk in health is our mind. Your mind is an environment of its own. You must avoid atmosphere of doubt or unbelief if you want to walk in health. A doubt-filled mind robs one of divine health.

You have to believe without any iota of doubt that you have been healed over 2,000 years ago by the stripes of Jesus Christ (Isaiah 53:5). Pay attention to your body, mind and physical surroundings. Stay clear from habits that are destructive to your body, guard your mind against doubt and ensure a clean and hygiene environment.

When you do, you glorify God, and He will keep sickness and diseases far from you. That is how to maintain the right environment for living in divine health.

KEY #14: N – NOTICE AND STOP YOUR NEGATIVE THOUGHTS

Did you know that what you think can either be beneficial to your walk in divine health or it can become a great hindrance? Your thoughts can affect how you feel and your life experiences. Your present state and estate is a direct result of your consistent thoughts pattern in the past. One of the keys to living in divine health is to consciously notice and stop your negative thoughts. Negative thoughts produce poor health.

Most of the severe panic attacks and spikes in blood pressure that people suffer were initiated solely by thoughts. Faith produces a healthy life, fear and anxiety produce depression, stress and illness. Your thoughts can change your brain, your cells and gene and keep you healthy or sick.

"As we think, we change the physical nature of our brain. As we consciously direct our thinking, we can wire out toxic patterns of thinking and replace them with healthy thoughts." – Dr. Caroline Leaf.

What most people who are up one day and down the next day need is a shift in the way they think. You want to change your life? Change your thinking! Change your thinking and you will be amazed as an entirely new life of health, beauty, prosperity, and continuous victory unfolds.

Are you experiencing poor health? It probably has nothing to do with your diet and lifestyle, but what goes on in between your ears. You have to consciously notice and stop your negative thoughts.

One of the strategies the devil uses to afflict people's health is to project thoughts of illness to them. He knows that you are what you think. If he can get you to dwell on thoughts of illness, you will soon manifest illness. That is why the Bible advises us never to confess sickness (Isaiah 33:24), but to confess what God has done for us through Christ Jesus. You must believe and confess that you have been healed to walk in divine health (Isaiah 53:5).

Every thought you think causes your brain to release neurotransmitters through which your brain communicates with your nervous system. The neurotransmitters control how your body function, from release of hormones to feeling of happiness, sadness, stress, anxiety or even digestion. Positive thoughts produce good health, negative thoughts lead to poor health.

Do not allow the devil influence your thoughts, resist him and he will flee from you (James 4:7). You must wage war against negative thoughts by ensuring you notice and stop your negative thoughts.

"Casting down imaginations, and every high thing that exalteth itself against the knowledge of God, and bringing into captivity every thought to

the obedience of Christ" (2 Corinthians 10:5).

What you perceive to be real becomes your physical reality. If you want a life of health, prosperity and constant victory, focus your thought on them. The Bible, our manual for successful living tells us how to think in Philippians 4:8. Think on:

> *"whatsoever things are true, whatsoever things are honest, whatsoever things are just, whatsoever things are pure, whatsoever things are lovely, whatsoever things are of good report; if there be any virtue, and if there be any praise, think on these things."*

So, there you have it, to live in divine health, you have got to see yourself living in divine health, in your mind's eyes. You must confess that you walk in divine health, your word when aligned to God's word produces tremendous results. Use your mouth to produce what you want.

KEY #15: O – OPPOSE THE DEVIL

Satan also known as the devil is not a mere metaphor, vague creature or nebulous concept but a real being. He is a real person with evil or dark powers. He is also a thief and his "purpose is to steal and kill and destroy" (John 10:10).

If you let the devil, he will steal your health from you, kill your joy and destroy everything in and around you. But you must not give him room in your life. One of the keys to living in divine health is to stand your ground against the devil. You must oppose the devil and fight his attempts to impose sickness on you.

The Bible tells the story of how Jesus healed a woman who was bent completely forward and was utterly unable to straighten herself up or to look upward for eighteen years in Luke 13:16. After Jesus healed her, some criticized Him for healing her on the Sabbath. In reaction to their criticism, Jesus said,

"Ought not this woman, being a daughter of Abraham, whom Satan hath bound, lo, these eighteen years, be loosed from this bond on the Sabbath day?"

Jesus made it clear that Satan was behind her afflictions.

This shows that many sickness and diseases people suffer is from the devil. The devil is the one who often oppress people with illness.

This does not in any way imply that every sickness is an affliction from the devil. While sickness most of the time is the result of living in a fallen world, it can also result from our actions and decisions or from environmental factors. Sickness can also result from a lifestyle of sin. This doesn't not mean that anyone sick is a sinner or under some curse.

It is important to however make it clear that sickness itself is a curse (Deuteronomy 28:61) and should never be entertained. And though Satan may not be the direct cause of every sickness, he is behind the fall of man. Sickness is a curse traceable to sin (the fall of man), and since Satan is the author of sin, he is indirectly or directly the agent of sickness.

Are you battling with a health condition? Are you desperately in need of healing? Are you tired of being up today and down tomorrow? Do you want to live in divine health? If you answered yes, get ready to fight the good fight of faith. Maybe you have been crying and asking God to heal you or chase the devil out of your life, stop!

The Bible says you have been healed already in Isaiah 53:5. And in James 4:7, the Bible made it clear that you are the one who is supposed to overcome the devil. How? To receive your healing, all you need do is believe that by the stripes of Jesus you have been healed over 2,000 years ago, and you must confess with your mouth that you are healed (1Peter 2:24, Romans 10:9 – 10). Then you need to stand your ground and rebuke the devil out of your life. Stand up against him and every symptoms of sickness with the Word of God.

"Submit yourselves therefore to God. Resist the devil and he will flee from you" (James 4:7).

One of the reasons God sent Jesus was for your healing. Healing is in Christ' Atonement. Jesus already came and is gone to be with the Father. He is not going to heal your today, He already did over 2,000 years ago. Receive your healing today by faith. Your body is the temple of the Holy Spirit, not sickness, so don't accommodate sickness in your body.

Whenever you notice any symptoms of sickness in your body, rebuke it and the devil behind it immediately using God's Word. That is how to oppose the devil and one of the keys to living in divine health.

KEY #16: P – PROSPEROUS SOUL

Health and wholeness is the will of God for all His children. God wants us well in every area of our lives. God wants us to prosper mentally, because our health, financial and physical prosperity depends on it. So, one of the keys to living in divine health is a prosperous soul (mind, will and emotions).

"Beloved, I wish above all things that thou mayest prosper and be in health, even as thy soul prospereth" (3 John 1:2).

The key to living in divine health and receiving physical and financial prosperity is found in the last part of the 3 John 1:2 verse, "even as your soul prospers". The Lord wants us to prosper our soul by receiving, meditating upon, believing in, and acting on His word. When we do, we will enjoy increased health, vitality and all round prosperity.

Good health and all round prosperity are the outward manifestations of a prosperous inner man (soul). Until you are prosperous and healthy on the inside, there will be no outward manifestation of prosperity and divine health.

Do you want to live in divine health? If so, you have got to live in divine health from the inside, and eventually, your health will be visible for all to see to the glory of God.

The inward unseen prosperity of the soul (the mind, will and emotions) is what produce the outward seen natural prosperity (health and success). If you ever want to live in divine health, commit to believing and acting on God's word, especially His word on divine health. A prosperous soul equals a healthy and prosperous man.

KEY #17: Q – QUIT EATING UNHEALTHY AND JUNK FOOD

Quit eating unhealthy and junk food if you want to live in health and lead an enjoyable and active life. One of the keys to living in divine health is to avoid food that causes fatigue, fluctuations of blood sugar level, memory impairment, and increased risk of liver, kidney and heart disease and other host of health problems related to nutrition.

Food is a blessing from God and we must receive it with gratitude.

"That each of them may eat and drink, and find satisfaction in all their toil – this is the gift of God" (Ecclesiastes 3:13).

Though food is a gift from God, it does not bring us near Him or separate us from Him.

"Food does not bring us near to God; we are no worse if we do not eat, and no better if we do" (1 Corinthians 8:8).

We need food on daily bases; we need food to stay alive and healthy, we need food to celebrate, to morn, to show affection, to care for people and for entertainment. The problem is in the quality and quantity of food we consume.

"Has thou found honey? Eat so much as is sufficient for thee, lest thou be filled therewith, and vomit it" (Proverbs 25:16).

There are several dangers of over-eating (gluttony) or

under-eating.

> *"It is not good to eat too much of honey..." (Proverbs 25:27). "Therefore I urge you to take some food. For it will give you strength..." (Acts 27:34 ESV).*

Eating unhealthy and junk food on a regular bases may also contribute to health problems. Watch what you eat. Your body is the temple of the Holy Spirit, don't destroy it with poor nutrition.

> *"I am allowed to do anything – but not everything is good for you. And even though 'I am allowed to do anything; I must not become a slave to anything" (1 Corinthians 6:12 NLT).*

Do you want to live daily in health? The key to living in divine health is to quit eating unhealthy and junk food. Junk food are any food that is highly processed and which is high in added sugar, salt and saturated fats.

Unhealthy and junk food contribute to the risk of developing some health problems like obesity, tooth decay, high blood pressure, high cholesterol, heart disease and stroke, depression, some cancers, osteoporosis, type-2 diabetes, eating disorder, etc.

Avoid food that make you sick, tired and even ineffective in the pursuit of your life given purpose and destiny. Instead, focus on good variety of healthy food from the five food groups each day. Eat more of fruits and vegetables. Eat sugar and fatty or salty food only occasionally and ensure you drink fresh clean water instead of sugary drinks. It is even better to cook your meal with healthy recipes that look and taste good.

Food is a gift from God and you are free to each whatever you like, but remember that with freedom comes responsibility. To live in divine health, eat wisely. Above all, remember that you are a spirit with a soul living in a body. As you feed your body with food, ensure your spirit is connected to Spirit of God through Christ Jesus and that your soul is well fed with the word of God.

KEY #18: R – REGULAR FASTING AND HOW IT AFFECTS HEALTH

One of the reasons most people hardly fast on regular basis is because they see fasting as what they stand to lose rather than what they stand to gain. God will not expect us to fast if it has no benefit.

Regular fasting is one of the keys to living in divine health. Jesus speaking in Matthew 6: 16 – 17, said, "When you fast". Notice that He didn't say, "If you fast", which means that God expects us to fast. It is a matter of when and not if.

What is fasting and how does it affect our health? Fasting is abstinence from food and drinks for a set period of time in order to give oneself totally to prayer and study of God's word. God promise healing and health to anyone who will fast according to His standard. Fasting goes beyond abstinence from food. Let see the kind of fasting God expects from us, the kind that guaranteed healing and health.

"Is not this the fast that I have chosen? To lose the bands of wickedness, to undo the heavy burdens, and to let the oppressed go free, and that ye break every yoke? Is it not to deal thy bread to the hungry, and that thou bring the poor that are cast out to thy house? When thou seest the naked, that thou cover him; and that thou hide not thyself from thine own flesh? Then shall

they light break forth as the morning, and thine health shall spring forth speedily: and thy righteousness shall go before thee; the glory of the Lord shall be thy reward" (Isaiah 58: 6 – 8).

When you fast, God's own way, God is committed to keeping you in divine health. God's recommended fasting is a guaranteed key to living in divine health.

<u>Here are ten Biblical reasons to fast:</u>

1. Fasting guarantees divine health and minister to the needs of others (Isaiah 58: 5 – 8).

2. Christ fasted and He expects us to fast too (Matthew 4:2, 6: 16 – 18).

3. Fasting helps us get guidance from God on what we should do and how (Acts 14:23, Judges 20: 26 – 28).

4. To show humility in the presence of God (Psalms 35:13).

5. For spiritual strength. Jesus fasting before commencing His earthly ministering. He fasted for spiritual strength (Luke 4: 1 – 11).

6. To seek deliverance or protection from enemies or circumstances (2 Chronicles 20: 3 – 4).

7. To express concern for the work of God and for the progress of the Kingdom of God here on earth (Nehemiah 1 : 3 – 4).

8. To overcome temptations and dedicate yourself to God (Matthew 4: 1 – 11).

9. To express love and worship for God (Luke 2:37).

10. For intensity in prayer and to get a good testimony

before the enemies (Ezra 8: 21 – 23).

Apart from the Biblical importance to fast, science and research has proven that fasting helps our health and well-being.

<u>Here are ten benefits of fasting backed by science.</u>

1. Fasting boost cognitive performance.

2. Fasting helps protect you from obesity and related chronic diseases.

3. Fasting during chemotherapy jump-start the immune system and exposes the cancer cell, thus ridding the body of old, toxic cells and replacing them with new healthy ones.

4. Regular fasting promotes blood sugar control by reducing insulin resistance.

5. It also helps fight inflammation thus promoting better health.

6. Fasting increases growth hormone secretion which is important for growth, metabolism, muscle strength and weight loss.

7. Fasting enhances heart health by improving cholesterol level and blood pressure.

8. Fasting promotes longevity.

9. Fasting improves your immune system

10. Regular fasting also improves eating patterns.

There you have it, the spiritual and scientific benefits of fasting. Do you want perfect and total health? One of the keys to living in divine health is regular fasting, when done properly.

KEY #19: S – SURPRISING CONNECTION BETWEEN SLEEP AND HEALTH

According to studies from the <u>Centers for Disease Control and Prevention</u>, sleep deprivation is epidemic.

The Bible speaking on the importance of sleep says in Psalms 127:2,

"It is vain for you to rise up early, to sit up late, to eat the bread of sorrows: for so he giveth his beloved sleep."

There is surprising connection between sleep and health. Getting enough sleep, between 7-8 hours a day, is one of the keys to living in divine health. Adequate sleep is essential for helping a person maintain vitality, optimal health and well-being.

Sleep is never a luxury. It is critical for your well-being. It helps your body function normally and naturally repair itself. Not getting enough sleep, over time leads to serious health problems or worsen some health problems. If you really want to live in divine health, ensure you sleep 7-8 hours every day.

Here are some surprising connections between sleep and health, and reasons to get more sleep.

1. God created you to need sleep:

You will malfunction when you don't sleep enough. Lack of adequate sleep affects us physically and emotionally. It can lead to frustration, stress and affects our ability to think creatively.

2. Lower rate of heart disease:

Getting enough sleep each night helps the body's blood pressure to regulate itself and reduce the risk of sleep-related health conditions such as apnea and help improve your heart health.

3. Prevent depression:

Many research link sleep disorder such as insomnia to high rate of depression and suicide.

4. Sharper brain:

Quality sleep help our memory. It helps the brain to focus and take in new information.

5. Immune system:

Lack of adequate sleep slows down the rate at which the immune cells attack foreign bodies and opens the body up for sickness more often.

While adequate sleep is good for your health, too much of it may do more harm than good. Your best bet is 7-8 hours of sleep each day for optimal health benefits.

KEY #20: T – TESTIMONIES ABOUT MIRACLE HEALING

Testimonies can have a very powerful effect upon those in desperate need of encouragement and God's intervention. The Bible speaking in Psalm 22:22 says,

"I will praise you to all my brothers; I will stand up before the congregation and testify of the wonderful things you have done."

Testimonies beget testimonies. God is no respecter of man, you can trust Him to do for you what He did for others. What He did yesterday, He can do today. Only believe!

Here are some testimonies of God's healing power to build your faith.

HIV/Aids Swallowed Up In Victory:

It all started in 2010 after feeling a strange sickness, I went for a medical check-up and I was confirmed HIV positive. Since that time, I have believed God for my total healing. I read books of Papa, The Healing Balm and the Miracle Meal and could minister the communion to myself often; serving in the sanctuary keeping unit, always attended Covenant Hour of Prayer and engaged passionately in Kingdom advancement prayers in my closet. Light dawned on me when

I heard the testimony of a sister who shared how God healed her of this deadly disease in Shiloh 2017. I knew God was up to something. I therefore made up my mind that the forthcoming year being my year of New Dawn, it should be evident in my health. I stopped at nothing as when the 21 days prayer and fasting started, I participated fully disregarding the strong drugs I was taking believing God for His grace to be sufficient for me.

To the glory of God, when I went for my medical appointment after prayer and fasting on February 23rd 2018, the doctor told me the machine could not detect the virus anymore in my blood and I shouted a resounding Hallelujah. Today, I am here to witness the healing power of God in this commission. I am now HIV-free.

CHANDIA JULIET

Source: https://www.winnerschapelughelli.com.ng/testimonies.php

COVID-19 Patient healed in Italy:

He had been a healthy athlete, a runner. All that changed when Luca* was diagnosed with COVID-19, which has put the entire globe in a tailspin the past few weeks. In the midst of recovery, Luca found himself growing antsy and impatient outside one of the wards at Samaritan's Purse Emergency Field Hospital in Cremona, Italy.

Stationed at the tent hospital in Italy, Jason and Damaris Scalzi, a chaplain couple from New Jersey, talked with Luca alongside an interpreter. He offered to pray with him to receive Christ. As Luca learned more, he wanted to accept Jesus Christ as his Savior. Days afterward, Luca was released from the hospital, healed from both spiritual and physical sickness.

Source: https://billygraham.org/story/powerful-moment-of-healing-with-covid-19-patient-in-italy/

Completely healed of strange ailment:

I thank God for preserving the life of my daughter. She suddenly became sick and started stooling continuously. I thank God for his intervention and for saving her life. She is completely healed of the strange ailment. I also got healed during the 2017 Prayer Conference of pain in my waist. – Sis Patricia Dominic

Source: https://rccgopenheavens.org/testimonies/

Before Surgery:

Hi, my name is Pat. I was having this excruciating pain that was in my back. It was like um one of the most miserable feelings, never having had that feeling before. I was nauseous. Anything that I ate, anything at all I had such pain in my midsection. I was at the point that even drinking water hurt my midsection.

So, my doctor, she said, I think we need to order an ultrasound of your gallbladder. And we got the results back and she called me. She said, "Your gallbladder is full of gallstones."

And she made an appointment with a surgeon and I was going to meet with him on July 3rd. On July 3rd, I had the appointment at like 9:30 in the morning so I was in, getting ready. I was watching 700 Club.

And then they said that they were going to pray. I just felt that I needed to stop getting ready. So, I went and stood in front of the TV with my hand on my abdomen and just as I started to pray.

Gordon says, "Someone else with deep pain in your abdomen from gallstones and a gallbladder condition, and God has healed that. He's taken away all the pain, all that infection. All the stones now in Jesus name be gone and be made whole."

And I'm telling you, the pain I had felt now for like two or three weeks, it was instantly gone. And I think, it's like, that's faith. I knew. I knew in my– in my knower, that the Lord had healed me.

And when the girl was doing the ultrasound, she said, Let me tell you, I can't find one stone in this gallbladder. And I went, Yes! Praise you, Jesus! It's just proof.

And so, my doctor comes walking in with his face beaming and he's holding up a paper and he said, You were so right. What was there is no longer there.

And I am doing wonderful. How do you explain the magnitude of a God that heals? He made these bodies and He knows how to fix them. And I'm very thankful to Him for the healing. It's the power of the Holy Spirit and I'm so appreciative.

Source: https://www1.cbn.com/video/WOK399v2/healed-right-before-surgery?show=700club

Crohn's Disease Healed:

On October 18, 2011 I attended a Full Gospel Business Men's dinner where Bruce Van Natta was speaking. I am so glad I attended that night, as a miracle occurred for me. He prayed a group prayer for everyone in the room that night and I was healed of Crohn's disease which I had been dealing with since the age of 13. I am 31 years old now and finally—my stomach feels whole again. Thank you God for my healing.

Thank you, Renata Steltman.

Source: https://sweetbreadministries.com/amazing-testimonies/

Healed of Ankle Pain:

French BSSM student wrote this testimony from his mission trip to South Africa:

One of my favorite moments of the trip to South Africa was the last night we were there. A group of us went to do a service at a church. At the end, during the ministry time, a friend asked me to pray with her for a young girl, who was about 13–14 years old. She had hurt her ankle doing gymnastics.

The doctor said it was going to take six weeks to recover, and she was in a lot of pain and couldn't even be with her friends. We prayed once and asked her to check her ankle pain and movement capacity. The pain decreased, but it was still there and painful. We prayed a second time. She took her flip-flop off and started to walk slowly. She turned back to walk back toward us and her parents, and she just exploded into tears and ran into her mom's arms and said,

"I am healed! All the pain left! I am healed! "

She was crying so much because of how happy and thankful she was for her miracle! This precious moment really touched me. He's better than we think. God doesn't need experts; He needs people that say yes.

Source: https://www.bethel.com/testimonies/healed-of-ankle-pain/

You are next on the line for a miracle

It does not matter what health condition you have, there is no illness or disease God cannot healed. Trust God's word for your healing.

God has already made provision for your healing. "But he was wounded for our transgressions, he was bruised for our iniquities: the chastisement of our peace was upon him; and with his stripes we are healed" (Isaiah 53:5). Receive your healing now, in Jesus' Name.

KEY #21: U – UNHEALTHY HABITS TO QUIT OR AVOID

To live in divine health, there are habits you must avoid or quit. These habits could harm your health and well-being. Paying attention to and correcting or avoiding harmful unhealthy habits is one of the keys to living in divine health.

It is popularly believed that whatever you do consistently for 8 days becomes a habit and that it takes 21 days to change a habit. The first step to change any habit is to become aware of the habit. Becoming aware of unhealthy habit is necessary to initiate the change.

Some of the unhealthy habits are seemingly innocent thing we do on daily basis, and these seemingly harmless habit negatively impact our health, while others are obviously harmful.

Here are ten unhealthy habits to quit or avoid so you can live in divine health.

1. Drinking too much juice:
Drinking juice like orange juice which is rich in Vitamin C, Vitamin B and various antioxidant is actually a good

habit but the problem lies in drinking too much of it. Too much juice can cause tooth decay, type 2 diabetes and obesity because of the high level of fructose (Proverbs 23:20).

2. Drinking alcohol excessively:

Abuse of alcohol leads to addictions and all sorts of health problems. (Proverbs 23:21, Galatians 5:21).

3. Sleeping for too long:

Sleeping 7-9 hours a day is recommended for an average adult. While too little sleep is unhealthy, sleep too much does much more harm. It increases the risk of diabetes, heart disease and stroke (Proverbs 6:9).

4. Skipping breakfast:

The habit of skipping meals regularly, especially breakfast can have trickle effect, and can affect your health and well-being. When your body lack food, it begins to conserve energy and burn fewer calories. This leads to sluggishness and reduced concentration and alertness. (Acts 27:34 ESV).

5. Avoid unhealthy and junk food:

Avoid any food that can cause fatigue, fluctuations of blood sugar level, memory impairment, and increased risk of health, kidney and liver problems, as well as health problems like high blood pressure, high cholesterol, stroke, depression, etc. (1 Corinthians 6:12)

6. Not drinking enough water:

It is recommended that we drink six to eight glasses of liquids such as water, juice, tea, etc. a day. Not drinking enough water can cause dehydration which can lead to health problems like constipation, headache, pile, muscle pain, etc. Drinking water help you feel more energized.

7. Smoking:

Smoking tobacco products of any kind does harm to both the smoker and people around him. Tobacco contain many toxic substances that poisons the body. This toxic substances can stop the central nervous system from functioning properly. Smoking can cause health issues such as shortness of breath, stomach ulcer, tooth bleeding, asthma, pneumonia, irritation of the vocal cord, increased risk of cancer, etc. (1 Corinthians 3:16-17).

8. Stress: avoid stress and anxiety like plagues:

An unhappy lifestyle can cause the release of stress hormones. These hormones can increase your sugar level, blood pressure, slow digestion, lower immunity and obesity. (Philippians 4:6).

9. Laziness and idleness:

Slothfulness slides the door open for sickness to enter. Productive work leads to a healthy life, laziness and idleness destroy the body. (Ecclesiastes 10:18).

10. Sinful lifestyle:

There was no sickness until man sinned in the Garden of Eden. Sin brought curse upon man, and in Deuteronomy 28:61, God listed sickness and diseases as curse. Every child of God is redeemed from curse and every sickness by Christ Jesus. However, when start living a sinful lifestyle, you open the door to curse, sickness and diseases in your life. (John 5:14).

These are just few habits that are unhealthy. If you want to live in divine health, avoid or quit every unhealthy habits.

KEY #22: V – VITALITY AT HOME

Regular exercise is necessary to keep fit, stay healthy and happy. Going to gym or hiring a workout instructor is optional as there are several exercises you can do at home. Vitality at home is one of the keys to living in divine health.

While exercising at a gym has a lot of benefits, some people prefer to exercise at home. Some of the reasons many people prefer exercising at home to visiting a gym are:

1. You can put on whatever you want to wear.

2. You only exercise when it is most convenient

3. It saves money

4. You can play your own music loud. You can combine exercising with listening to a great Gospel message or song.

5. You will be forced to educate yourself about exercise and fitness.

The bible recommends bodily (physical) exercise even though it places premium on spiritual exercise. Your body is a gift from God, you can't afford not to care for it. One of the ways to take care of the body is through regular exercise.

"For bodily exercise profiteth little: but godliness is profitable unto all

Do you want to live in divine health? Create time for bodily exercise. Here are some health benefits of regular exercise.

1. Exercise elevates your mood: Active exercise stimulates brain chemicals that make you feel great and lifts your mood.

2. Exercise might help you think more clearly: Research shows that regular exercise is good for cognitive function.

3. Exercise improves muscle strength: Keeping fit helps keep your muscles strong, joints, tendons and ligaments flexible, making it possible to more easily and avoid injury.

4. Exercise is good for your heart.

5. Regular exercise lowers your risk of developing type 2 diabetes.

6. It helps some people manage anxiety and depression.

7. Daily exercise helps promote restful sleep.

8. You can control your weight with exercise.

9. Regular exercise can reduce some of the effects of ageing.

10. Keeping fit enhances your immune system.

Vitality at home is the secret of longevity and a healthy life. Below are some of the exercises to try out at home:

1. Press-up

2. Dumbbell standing shoulder press

3. Skipping

4. Dumbbell squat

5. Bench dips

6. Crunch

7. Shadow boxing

8. Wall sit

9. Squat Reach and Jump

10. Single and double Leg Abdominal Press, etc.

Why spend money visiting a gym when there's the living room floor? Well, it's a matter of preference. Start exercising today, keep fit, say healthy.

KEY #23: W – WHY WORK IS GOOD FOR OUR HEALTH

Work is a blessing and not a curse. God is the inventor of work. Before the fall of man at the Garden of Eden, God assigned Adam and Eve to the important work of cultivating the garden.

Work existed before man sinned, disobedience that brought the whole of humanity under sin's curse. So work couldn't have been a punishment for man's disobedience. Work is God's original design for man.

"The Lord God took the man and put him in the garden of Eden to work it and keep it." (Genesis 2:15 ESV.)

The truth is that man was designed to find fulfillment in work. We are stewards of God's creation through our work. Even God worked so hard to create the universe, He worked so hard that He needed to take some rest. If work is evil, God would not have worked, because He is infinitely good and does not associate with evil.

"And on the seventh day God ended his work which he had made; and he rested on the seventh day from all his work which he had made." (Genesis 2:2)

Work is good and it is one of the keys to living in divine health. Work is good for our health and well-being. Why is work good for our health? Here are just few reasons why work is good for our health.

1. Laziness and idleness destroys the body. "By much slothfulness the building decayeth; and through idleness of the hands the house droppeth through." idleness causes the body (building/temple of God) sick (decay). If you want to live in divine health, you must work.

2. An idle mind is the devils workshop. Laziness and idleness leads to sin, sin brings curse, including sickness and diseases. (Read John 5:14).

3. Work leads to longevity. And that is why most people die few years after retirement. God created us to work. If you stop working, you start dying. You could be retired from your paid job, but never retire from work.

4. It is a proven fact that those who work enjoy happier and healthier lives than those who do not work.

5. Work increases recovery from illness. Those who lie down on the bed when ill remain sick for long, because work improves physical and mental health and aids quicker recovery from sickness.

If you want to live in divine healthy, find something useful to get engaged in. Work is not a curse. It is how we make our lives count and enrich our lives and that of others.

KEY #24: X – X-RAY YOUR LIFE AND WORDS

Until your soul is prosperous, you won't be in health. If you want to live in divine health, your heart must be renewed. You have got to think like God, act like God and talk like Him. You have got to let God's word rule your heart and influence your words.

"Keep thy heart with all diligence; for out of it are the issues of life." (Proverbs 4:23).

You cannot walk in divine health confessing and claiming sickness. Be careful what you say because you may have it.

"Death and life are in the power of the tongue: and they that love it shall eat the fruit thereof." (Proverbs 18:21).

Just like an X-Ray, the word of God helps us see through the outside to see exactly what's on our inside, and what needs to be fixed, so we can fix it.

"For the word of God is quick, and powerful, and sharper than any two-edged sword, piercing even to the dividing asunder of soul and spirit, and of the joints and marrow, and is a discerner of the thoughts and intents of the heart." (Hebrews 4:12).

God's word is alive, it is powerful, and a reveler of thoughts and intents of the heart. X-Raying our lives means to expose our heart to the influence of the word. Your mouth speaks what is in your heart. When you heart is saturated with faith-filled scriptures on divine healing, your mouth will voice them out, and your body will have no choice but to align. That is how to renew your mind.

We must meditate on God's word so we can know what is ours and seize it by faith. If you don't know what is yours, it will elude. Many people are battling with illness because they are ignorant of the fact that Jesus has healed them (Isaiah 53:5).

If you are finding it difficult to walk in divine health, you are up today and down tomorrow, you need to X-Ray your life with the word of God to reveal where the problem is coming from. It is not enough to believe you have been healed, you must prove it through your words and action.

"Talk no more so exceeding proudly; let not arrogancy come out of your mouth: for the Lord is a God of knowledge, and by him actions are weighed."1 Samuel 2:3).

Your health is tied to the prosperity of your soul. Until you are healthy on the inside, you won't be healthy on the outside. Soul prosperity is only possible through constant mediation on the word and by allowing the word to influence your thoughts and words.

"This book of the law shall not depart out of thy mouth; but thou shalt meditate therein day and night, that thou mayest observe to do according to all that is written therein: for then thou shalt make thy way prosperous, and then thou shalt have good success." (Joshua 1:8).

You X-Ray your life and word with God's word. The more you expose yourself to the word, the more your life is transformed according to God's will. God's will is that you prosper and be in health.

The enemies of divine health, such as sin, ignorance, weak faith and personal disobedience are destroyed when exposed to the influence of God's word.

"All scripture is given by inspiration of God, and is profitable for doctrine, for reproof, for correction, for instruction in righteousness" (2 Timothy 3:16).

One of the keys to walking in divine health is to X-Ray your life and word with God's word. You are not permitted to confess what you don't like. Speak what you want into being.

"And the inhabitant shall not say, I am sick: the people that dwell therein shall be forgiven their iniquity." (Isaiah 33:24).

Never confess that you are sick, rather say, "By the stripes of Jesus, I have been healed and I am healed forever". Say it and believe because God said so

KEY #25: Y – YOU ALWAYS HAVE A CHOICE

You have a will, and with your will you can choose to live in divine health. The point is that you always have a choice. God will not override your freedom of choice. If you decide to die sick or poor or a failure, God will not stop you. He has set before your life and death, and He has advised you to choose life so it will be well with you, but it is your responsibility to make that choice.

"I call heaven and earth to record this day against you, that I have set before you life and death, blessing and cursing: therefore choose life, that both thou and thy seed may live" (Deuteronomy 30:19).

We have been looking at the keys to living in divine health, it is up to you to take these keys seriously or to discard them. Just like Salvation, God has made healing and divine health available to everyone. Salvation is available to everybody but not everyone is saved. Only those who accept Jesus as their Lord and Savior became born again (saved). That is how it is with healing and divine health. Though healing and divine health is available to all, many are afflicted by one sickness or the other. You have to receive your healing and make up your mind to walk in divine health. It like FM radio signal, though it is available in your room, but you still have to tune to the right frequency to listen to the radio station.

There are those who erroneously beg God to heal them. But that is not scriptural, because the Bible makes is clear that God has already sent Jesus for your healing. He has made provisions for you to walk in divine health. By the stripes of Jesus, you have been healed (1 Peter 2:24). It is now your responsibility to believe and receive what is yours. And you receive through faith, not by crying and begging God.

Faith always please God, and our faith for healing and divine health must be on God's word and not on what we do. There are people who exercise regularly, eat healthy food, live in clean environment, sleep 7 -9 hours daily, avoid stress like plague and visit doctors regularly for check-up, yet they are always battling with one illness or the other. It is not faith in what we do, but the word of God that guarantees divine health.

The word of God never fails, and it is your responsibility to make the Word work for you. Unfortunately, no one can do that for you. I can expose you to what the word of God says about healing and divine health, but it is you that must make the Word work for you. No one will do your believing for you, you must do your believing.

"The just must live by his faith" (Habakkuk 2:4). It must be by your own faith.

Do you want to live in divine health all the days of your life, it your choice to make. Remember you always have a choice. I have presented you with the keys to living in divine health, read them over and over again, look up the scriptural quotations, and meditate on them over and over until the word of God on divine health comes alive in you, only then can you manifest divine health.

KEY #26: Z – ZION, A PLACE OF ABSOLUTE HEALTH

The last and the most important of all the keys to living in divine health is to be translated into Zion, a place of absolute health. To dwell in Zion, you must be born again. When we got born again, we were born into Zion. That is where we currently reside and live spiritually. We are citizens of Zion already, and it is a place of total and absolute health.

"But ye are come unto mount Sion, and unto the city of the living God, the heavenly Jerusalem, and to an innumerable company of angels, to the general assembly and church of the firstborn, which are written in heaven, and to God the judge of all, and to the spirits of just men made perfect, and to Jesus the mediator of the new covenant, and to the blood of sprinkling, that speaketh better things than that of Abel." (Hebrews 12:22-24).

Notice that Bible didn't say we shall come to mouth Zion. It said we are already in Zion, the city of the living God. We live and operate from Zion, spiritually. Do not forget that you are a spirit with a soul living in a body. You must learn to operate from your spirit. Until you operate from your reborn human spirit, you will live a life lesser than what God destined for you.

There is a way of living and talking in Zion. And you can

learn to live and talk that way by renewing your mind. Remember that only your human spirit got born again, not your mind. That is why your mind must be renewed with the world of God. Until you do, there will be no difference between you and the man who is not saved.

Unless you renew your mind, you will not be able to prove what is good, acceptable, and perfect, will of God.

"And be not conformed to this world: but be ye transformed by the renewing of your mind, that ye may prove what is that good, and acceptable, and perfect, will of God" (Romans 12:2). You must learn the vocabularies of Zion.

It is forbidden to say I am sick in Zion. In Zion, we don't confess feeling but the word of God. It doesn't matter what you feel, what the doctors have said, what matters in Zion is what the word of God says. The word of God said we have been healed by the stripes of Jesus, which is what we believe and confess.

When you hear someone say "I am sick", the person is either ignorant or does not belong to Zion. In Zion, we confess what we want, and what we want is what the word of God says is ours.

"And the inhabitant shall not say, I am sick: the people that dwell therein shall be forgiven their iniquity" (Isaiah 33:24).

Are you a citizen of Zion? Are you born again? It will be impossible to live in divine health if you have not accepted Jesus as your Lord and Savior. You can receive Jesus into your heart even now. If you will like to make Jesus you Lord, <u>click here to pray the prayer of salvation</u>.

The end of A-Z of Divine Health!

Thank you for reading my book. If you enjoyed it, won't you please take a moment to leave me a review at your favorite retailer?
Thanks!
Chidi Anslem Adim
info@chidianslem.com

ABOUT THE AUTHOR

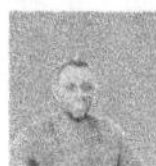

Chidi Anslem Adim is a Gospel minister with The Redeemed Christian Church of God. Curr ently serving as the minister in charge of the youth's ministry, RCCG Ambassador's house, Port Harcourt and the head of prayer and media departments. He is a graduate of Electrical and Electronics Engineering, a sort after inspirational and motivational speaker and a Gospel blogger.

He is the author of "The End of Sickness: Go beyond healing to living a sickness free life!" He is happily married, with a thriving family.

Anslem's vision is to share God's love and the life-transforming messages of the Bible with the world. He has a public diary of his thoughts and teachings at www.chidian slem.com

OTHER BOOKS BY CHIDI ANSLEM ADIM

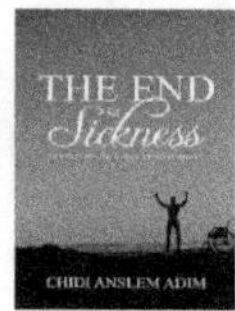

In this brief, but thorough Bible-based study, Anslem proves to you that healing is God's will for you. In this book, you will discover where sickness comes from, why many Christians still get sick, 10 lies of Satan people believe about divine healing, the truth about Paul's thorn in the flesh, how to receive your healing and how to keep your healing so you can go beyond healing to living a sickness free life.

ISBN: 978-1-00521-053-3 (ebook), ISBN: 979-8-66001-083-5 (paperback). Available At Your Favorite Stores. For more information and sample chapters, email info@chi dianslem.com

www.ingramcontent.com/pod-product-compliance
Lightning Source LLC
Chambersburg PA
CBHW071225240726
48654CB00009B/928